ROADMAP TO A SUCCESSFUL MATCH: A RESIDENT'S PERSPECTIVE

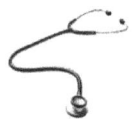

Dallas Wright, D.O.

Contribution from
Tyrone Philipson, M.D., EMT-P

Copyright © 2014 MedEmbark

All rights reserved. No part of this publication may be reproduced, stored in a retrieval system, or transmitted in any form or by any means, electronic, mechanical, photocopying, recording or otherwise, without the prior written permission of the author.

Disclaimer
The material in this book is for educational purposes only. Although the author and publisher have taken reasonable effort to ensure that the information in this book was current and accurate at the time of publication, the author and publisher do not assume and hereby disclaim any liability to any party for any loss, damage or disruption caused by errors or omissions, whether such errors or omissions result from negligence, accident, or any other cause. The views expressed by the individuals in this book do not necessarily reflect the views by their employers and/or affiliated organizations. Readers are encouraged to confirm the information contained herein with other sources as the process of advancing from medical student to resident is highly complex.

Printed in the U.S.A

ISBN-10: 0692390480
ISBN-13: 978-0-692-39048-1

Introduction

Congratulations on entering the next phase of your career development. This is an exciting time in your life. The transition from medical student to resident is filled with many uncertainties. The goal of this book is to highlight those uncertainties and assist you in your professional development. This book will not address the match process in its entirety. Instead, it will focus on key areas of concern typically found among medical students. Although the majority of this book is tailored to emergency medicine candidates, the ideas presented and discussed can be applied across many specialties. Keep in mind that neither the selection process nor the value placed on the selection criteria is the same for all programs. I highly recommend you research each program to identify program specific information before applying the concepts in this book. Best of luck!

The best way to predict your future is to create it
— Abraham Lincoln

Regards
Dallas Wright, D.O.

Acknowledgments

Special thanks: To family and friends for supplying me with life's greatest gift.

...Hey fatboy!

– Dallas

Contents

Introduction ………………………………….i

Acknowledgements …………………………..ii

1. Have a Plan ..…………………………....1

2. Which Emergency Medicine
   Candidates Match? ………………….7

3. The Emergency Medicine Clerkship ….....12

4. Application (CV, Personal Statement,
   Letters of Recommendation) …………….18

5. The Interview …..……………………….30

6. After the Interview …..…………………38

7. International Medical Graduate
   Considerations …………………………..40

8. Final Words …………………………....48

Chapter 1

Have a Plan

The most important component to a successful match is having a development plan with goals. Ask any successful person and you'll probably hear a different strategy on how to become successful and why their strategy is superior to the last. The reality is the path to success is not the same for everyone. The underlining theme, however, is the same: If you know what you want, you are moving in the right direction.

To know exactly what you want requires a little soul searching. I know, it sounds miserable. It is much easier to memorize the entire Krebs cycle than get in touch with your inner self. But, taking the time to develop a plan on where you want to be in 10 years will have a huge impact when you are applying for residency, interviewing and ranking programs. The development plan doesn't have to be extensive and the goals can be high-level. Knowing your finish point gives you a target to aim at and makes developing your roadmap much easier.

To better understand your long term goals answer these questions:

1. Do you want to stay in academic medicine or go out into the community?

   How you define success will help you answer this question. For example, is your goal to become a program director, obtain a faculty position, pursue research, become an administrator, teach residents, nurses, EMTs, paramedics or medical students, work in a large institution, work at a small institution, work at a center with specialty coverage (ENT, Ophthalmology, OB/Gyn, etc.), pursue a fellowship, live close to family and friends or practice medicine abroad.

2. What program length do you need?

   There are clear differences between 3 year programs, 4 years programs and starting with a traditional rotating internship. Examples of these differences include research time, cost of living, family life, academic appointments, confidence level and maturity. I encourage you to research the differences between each of these and see which one aligns best with your long term goals. As the restrictions on resident work-hour tightens the length of certain programs will likely change. Luckily for now, you can still consider this option in your decision making.

3. Do you learn best in/from a busy, chaotic environment or a slow, fairly controlled environment?

   You will learn medicine no matter which type of program you choose. The environment in which you work will either help or hinder the process.

4. Do you have special interests beyond emergency medicine?

   Are you interested in EMS, wilderness medicine, air medical transport, critical care, forensic medicine, medical direction, obtaining an advanced degree (JD, PhD, MPH, etc.)? Some programs are more supportive than others. If you end up at a program that doesn't offer what you want, then create it. In this day and age, medicine is filled with opportunities. For many of us though, there is a natural tendency to not pursue certain interests because of the notion that, "it's not offered so I can't do it," or "only someone trained in that can do it." The reality is quite the opposite. History is filled with people who rose to the top and never received advanced training or a degree—I'm looking at you Bill Gates.

5. Are you being smart about your program choice?

Make sure the philosophy of the program aligns with your goals. For example, if you're applying to a program that is heavily involved in research, make sure you want the same level of involvement and tailor your CV accordingly (see the CV section in Chapter 4). Most programs will discuss their interests and accomplishments on their website. Spending a few minutes browsing through the website can give you an enormous amount of information and help you judge what they might be looking for in a candidate. If the website information is limited, then reach out to one of the current residents. A simple phone call or email can go a long way.

Successfully matching into a residency program is becoming more and more competitive. The Association of American Medical Colleges reported a total of 17,343 U.S. medical school graduates for the class of 2012. The total number increased to 18,156 for the class of 2013. The number of residency applications is also increasing. According to the National Resident Matching Program (NRMP), the total number of applicants registered for the 2014 Match reached an all-time high of 40,394. The number of emergency medicine applicants has also increased from 1,803 in 2012 to 2,061 in 2013.

What does this mean for you? If you have perfect board scores, are at the top of your class, graduating from a prestigious medical school, spend your free time helping underserved communities and play golf with the program director on Saturdays, probably nothing. But, if you are like the majority of average medical students and by "average", I mean very smart but due to the dehumanizing nature of the medical education system thought to be mediocre—you should pay close attention to a few things described below. This will increase your likelihood of success and help reduce your cost since you pay for an opportunity to be interviewed.

First, some programs offer interviews based on a scoring system. Meaning, you get a certain number of points depending on your class rank, board score, etc. So, if your application has a total of 50 points and the minimum number of points needed to be offered an interview is 51, you just donated money to that program. In addition, 54% of programs have a minimum cutoff USMLE step 1 score when considering interviews. Some programs only offer interviews to candidates that rotate at their institution. Knowing which programs function this way can help save you money and be ready for the expensive interview season.

Second, keep in mind that future employers are more interested in whether or not you are board certified than what residency program or medical school you attended. Who do you think is the smarter physician, a board certified emergency physician that graduated from Harvard University or a board certified emergency physician that graduated from the University of Texas Health Science center?

Additional questions to consider:

6. What choice is best for my family?
7. Will the geographical location work?
8. What perks does this program offer (professional membership dues, vacation, educational, elective days/stipend/books, opportunities, meals, laundry services, parking, sports facilities, etc.)?

Knowing your 10 year plan will help you answer these questions. The more detailed the plan the easier it is to answer the questions.

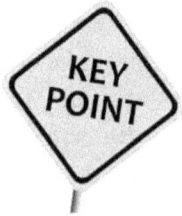

The most important component to a successful match is having a development plan with goals

Chapter 2

Which Emergency Medicine Candidates Match?

Trying to identify the key factors that correlate with success is challenging. When you ask most mentors they will tell you to "work hard," and "do well on the board exams." Fortunately, for the medical students with average grades and board scores there is much more to it than that.

Successfully matching in emergency medicine is a two-way street. The program matches to you and you match to the program. Each match has its own set of unique rules and criteria.

On the candidate matching side, studies evaluating factors impacting a candidate's decision and ultimate placement have been conducted. None of which have been very helpful. Most studies report friendliness, program personality, faculty enthusiasm, interview day, academics and geographical location as important to a candidate's program selection.

On the program matching side, multiple studies have tried to identify factors that impact the placement of a candidate on a program's rank list.

Most studies, not surprisingly, are filled with inconsistences. One study found that emergency medicine clerkship grades, medical school class rank and SLOE global assessment correlated with a higher placement on a program's rank list whereas, higher USMLE scores resulted in lower placement. Interestingly, none of these factors correlated with a candidate's overall position on the rank list. In another study, EM rotation grade, interview and clinical grades correlated better with program director selection criteria than Alpha Omega Alpha Honor Society (AOA) status, medical school attended, extracurricular activities, basic science grades, publications and personal statement.

The use of Electronic Residency Application Service (ERAS) does not change a program director's subjective rating of applicants. What is clear about ERAS is it makes submitting an application quick and easy. But, like swiping a credit card to pay for an item, you can quickly throw away money. As the number of applications submitted each year increases so does the work load of the administrator. This could lead to stricter filtering criteria in the future. Make sure you are serious about the programs before submitting an application.

As you can see, the key factors used to rank a

candidate are highly dependent on the program doing the ranking. This is why knowledge about the programs and their philosophy are so important.

Finally, do you know about the 9 P's? During an online interview with Michelle Lin, MD, Editor-in-Chief of Academic Life in Emergency Medicine, Dr. Gus Garmel, Stanford-Kaiser EM Residency Co-Program Director, discussed the impact of interview day and the 9 P's that program directors look for: performance, productivity, professionalism, personality, preparation, persistence, punctuality, passion and potential. Obviously, these cannot be fully assessed by paper alone. So keep them in mind when you are interviewing.

One truism is that program selection criteria does not change overnight. Therefore, having a clear understanding of which selection criteria a program uses will help you better understand your likelihood of matching at that program. Some programs will not offer you this information. Others will tell you exactly what they are looking for in a candidate.

A good place to start your detective work is with the current residents. First, they have just been through the match process. Second, each of them has something unique the program wants or needs. For example, do the majority of residents have interests in international medicine? Or, do most of the residents have EMS backgrounds? Obviously, the EMS background isn't what the program is looking for per se. Rather, it is the underlining qualities that someone with an EMS background possess including professionalism, team attitude, personal integrity, confidence, self-driven, etc. If you pay attention during casual conversations with residents you might identify key characteristics that the program finds valuable.

When discussing the program with a resident keep in mind that the PGY level of the resident will likely impact what he or she finds important. For example, when evaluating a potential candidate, a first year resident will probably put more emphasis on academic performance whereas, a senior resident may put more value on clinical experience and hands on demonstrations of knowledge. As residents advance through the various stages of education the factors they deem important change and mature.

What does it all mean? You are much more than a class rank and board score. Approximately 46% of programs are only interested in whether or not you passed step 1 of the USMLE (38% reported for COMLEX). For step 2 of the USMLE, 25% of programs are only interested in a passing score (29% reported for COMLEX). Failing the USMLE or COMLEX is extremely damaging. In the 2013 NRMP Program Director Survey, 77% of programs would seldom consider applicants who fail their USMLE Step 1 on the first attempt.

Even though class rank and board scores can determine whether or not you are offered an interview at certain programs, neither one reflects the important qualities unique to a great physician: professionalism, hard-working, being an active listener, sincere, humble, reliable, confident, calm, integrity, balanced, team leader, effective communicator, hunger for knowledge, etc. The more you know about a particular program the more accurately you can judge its suitability. Remember, information is power.

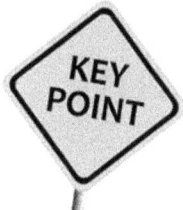 Having a clear understanding of which selection criteria a program uses will help you better understand your likelihood of matching at that program

Chapter 3

The Emergency Medicine Clerkship

This is not the time to figure out if emergency medicine is right for you. That decision should have been made when you created your professional development plan (see chapter 1). Instead, this is the time for you to identify the programs that will help you reach your goals. The hospitals you choose for your clerkships will ultimately depend on your goals. I would recommend researching the various types of training sites (large tertiary hospitals, community hospitals, small rural hospitals, etc.) and see which one makes sense for you. Keep in mind that you will see a wide range of disease pathology in emergency medicine. If you limit the number of emergency medicine clerkships in your 4th year to three you will have more time to learn about the various specialties (cardiology, ophthalmology, orthopedics, sports medicine, toxicology, radiology, OB/Gyn, etc.) and how to best approach these diseases. This will give you more knowledge and tools to prepare and enable you for the clerkship.

You must perform well in your clerkship to be considered for an interview. Receiving honors in the clerkship was cited by 80% of program directors as a factor in selecting applicants to interview. In order to perform well and stand out it is essential that you prepare for this rotation. In this day and age, not standing out will place you in the danger zone for not matching. Not performing well will surely set off red flags for the program director and ruin any chance of successfully matching at that institution.

Good preparation means you know the basics of common problems and issues in emergency medicine. Common problems are diabetic ketoacidosis, Myocardial Infarct, Acute Exacerbations of CHF/COPD/Asthma, GI bleeding, etc. Common issues are related to the various legal and ethical situations such as EMTALA, DNR, advance directives, etc.

The Society for Academic Emergency Medicine (SAEM) has a free emergency medicine primer that I encourage you to download and review. Although the breadth of knowledge required in emergency medicine is astonishing, making sure you brush up on the most common complaints prior to your clerkship will have a big impact.

First, most residents and attendings ask questions on topics they believe are important. As you can image, questions on HLA gene type and embryonic development do not usually make the list of "pimp" questions. Questions that do make the list typically focus on those aspects of patient care most concerning to the resident or attending. For example, "how should we correct this patient's serum sodium if it is 119mEq/L?"

Second, in a busy emergency department there is not much time for basic teaching. A firm understanding of the common problems and there management will demonstrate next level thinking and allow time to springboard into other conversations that give you valuable insight and information about the program. Even discussing general topics in emergency medicine, lifestyle and local activities can give you information about the program.

Not spending the time to prepare can have detrimental effects. The last thing a resident wants to do when he or she is behind in their work is spend 15 minutes explaining the basics of how to read an EKG. Don't get me wrong, most residents enjoy teaching and don't expect you to be an expert on EKG interpretation. But, knowing when to ask questions is important. Unfortunately, many medical students fail to recognize when it is a bad time to ask questions. When in doubt, write your questions down and ask the resident if he or she can discuss them with you when the shift is over.

Being an active learner is an important part of your clerkship. Reevaluating patients and staying current with laboratory results are good examples. Not only is it part of your education but you will be a superstar if you identify a critical finding the resident happened to miss. That being said, reporting every laboratory finding to the resident just to show him or her you are keeping up with the results is annoying. Having an enthusiastic medical student in the emergency department is refreshing. Just be careful not to overdo it. Maintaining a balance is the key.

A final thought on preparation is making sure to gather all the necessary information ahead of time. Knowing what is expected of you and how you are evaluated at the beginning of your clerkship will prevent a rocky start. The goal is to start strong and finish stronger. Ask for feedback at the end of each shift. It will demonstrate your desire to improve and is an easy way of leading into other potentially important conversations. You may get a few "tips" on how to impress certain attendings or who are the key decision makers.

You should have contact information handy on the student coordinator or residency coordinator. Make sure you have all the questions below answered prior to the start of your clerkship.

1. Where is the emergency department located?
2. What time does my shift start (arrive 15 minutes earlier)?
3. Where can I park?
4. Who am I meeting on the first day?
5. Did I complete all required paperwork (HIPPA, universal precautions, etc.)?
6. What dress attire/color scrubs should I wear?

7. Do I have my nametag/ID badge?
8. Do I have my stethoscope?
9. Do I have a smartphone/pocket book for quick referencing?
10. Do I have at least 2 pens (black ink)?
11. Do I have note paper?
12. Do I have a penlight?
13. Do I have trauma sheers?
14. Do I have a snack/lunch and water?
15. Do you know who the program director is?
16. Did I pack an interview outfit (if at an away rotation)?
17. Did I bring copies of my CV (if at an away rotation)?

We all know the importance of a first impression. Smile and introduce yourself to the residents and attendings. Always put your best foot forward. Just do not pretend to be someone you're not. Most physicians can spot a fake. Residency programs benefit from honesty just as much as you do. So just be you and everything else will fall into place.

It is important to realize that at this stage in your professional development you do not know who the decision makers are. For some programs, the residents determine how the candidates are ranked. At other programs, faculty members determine how candidates are ranked while at others, residents and faculty members rank candidates together. In my opinion, the best approach is to assume everyone is a decision maker. Even the nursing staff can influence whether or not you match. The emergency department is a close-knit team and how you perform spreads like wild fire. Be courteous to everyone. Do not let someone having a bad day ruin your chance of matching. Resist the urge to bad-mouth other programs or specialties. This includes emails and text messages. Always keep your persona positive.

After you've established a good rapport with the residents ask about their experience with interviews. Most of them have sat on the interview panel and can provide valuable information on how the process unfolds, pitfalls to avoid and help identify the decision makers.

Meet with the program and medical directors and introduce yourself to any faculty members you have not met before your clerkship has finished. Medical students with initiative will learn faster and discover more about the program and be seen by others as someone that acts and gets things done.

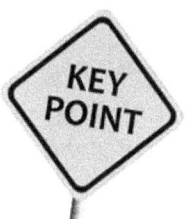

Good preparation and on-going hard work are the keys to performing well and standing out in your clerkship

Chapter 4

Application (CV, Personal Statement, Letters of Recommendation)

The application process in and of itself is fairly straight forward when using the Electronic Residency Application Service (ERAS). The upside is it's quick and easy. Typically you just "copy and paste" into the boxes provided. The downside is the final product often looks like a nine year-old put together your application. Fortunately, most residency programs are now familiar with the format.

The information you enter into the ERAS application is important. Resist using information from high school. The quickest way to tell a program you lack accomplishments is by adding high school awards to your application. Focus instead on the things you did in undergraduate, graduate and medical school. If you have any work experience, make sure you tailor it to the specialty you are applying to.

Start your application early. CV, personal statement and letters of recommendation should be ready by July of the application year. If you do not have all your letters of recommendation completed make sure you keep on top of the person writing them (tactfully of course). You do not want to find out he or she went on vacation before finishing your letter. Asking at the last minute for a letter of recommendation will not end well for you. You must have a completed application including all letters of recommendation to be offered an interview.

MyERAS opens to all applicants on July 1st. You can submit your completed applications for AOA programs and ACGME programs on July 15th and September 15th respectively. Apply as early as possible because interview slots are limited.

The programs you apply to should align with your developmental plan (refer to Chapter 1). The total number of programs you apply to depends on the overall strength of your application. In general, you should expect an interview offer from at least half of the total number of programs that receive your application. Historically, you have greater than 90% probability of matching if you are ranking more than 8 to 10 programs. The average number of programs ranked by a candidate that successfully matched in 2011 was 10.8.

The medical student performance letter (MSPL/Deans Letter) is an important part of your application and provides a statistical breakdown of your performance. Other than the unique characteristics section, you have little control over its content. So it will not be discussed here.

Curriculum Vitae (CV)

There is a great article, "So You Want a New Job: Time to Update Your CV," by Barbara Katz, Kevin M. Klauer, DO, FACEP and James G. Adams, MD, FACEP that covers the important aspects of creating a CV. Some of the information in this section will be drawn from that article. I encourage you to read it before finalizing your CV.

Complete your CV before you apply to residency. This will make filling out your application on ERAS easier. The number of programs that will ask you for a copy of your CV is small. However, you do not want to be the one applicant that was not prepared. So have a copy with you during the interview. Make sure you follow these considerations when crafting your CV:

1. Proof read, proof read, proof read. Then have someone else proof read.
2. Information should be in reverse chronological order starting with the most recent.
3. Organize your CV with information on the

left and dates on the right.
4. Make sure the time frame between jobs, education and activities are complete and accurate.
5. Start your CV with "Education" or "Training and Education." The order in which the remaining sections are arranged depends on your strengths and weaknesses. For example, if you worked as a pharmacist before medical school the next section could be "Professional Experience." If you have been recognized on multiple occasions for your academic achievements then "Honors & Awards" might come next. Choose wisely as you only have a few seconds to capture the reader's interest. Additional section heading examples include Professional Experience, Additional Work Experience, Certification & Licensure, Professional Activities, Honors & Awards, Research & Publications, Posters & Presentations, Academic Appointments & Committees, Professional Memberships.
6. Do not overdo the italics, bold text and underlines. Keep it clean and to at least font size 12.
7. The last section should be "Personal."

Hopefully, you have been updating your CV throughout medical school. If you have not, now is the time to review what you have and identify your weak areas (leadership experience, extracurricular activities, research, professional memberships, etc.).

Fill the gaps or have an action plan working towards filling those gaps. Remember that certain areas of the CV will be more important for some programs and less important to others. Make sure your CV aligns with your career goals.

In general, highlight your strengths and minimize your weaknesses. Content and format are equally important. Adding the "casting workshop" you did in the 2nd year of medical school may not be the best use of space on your CV. Add items instead that reflect why you are an accomplished leader, why you became fully involved in medical school and any distinctive factors that separate you from other candidates. See the CV example for ideas.

Personal Statement

The personal statement is your opportunity to give the reader a glimpse into who you truly are. I use the word "glimpse" because it should be no longer than one page. Do not put your CV in paragraph form and do not use the personal statement from your medical school application. The past 3 to 4 years should have enriched and broadened your outlook on the future. You are closing one chapter of your life and starting a new one. Remember your plan? Residency is the next step in your professional career development. How you write your personal statement depends on the message you are sending to the reader. Multiple studies have looked at the topics written in medical

Example CV

JOHN DOE

Street Address
City, State, Zip code
Phone number
email address

EDUCATION	DATE
Doctor of Medicine University of California, Irvine School of Medicine Irvine, CA	Expected 2014
Bachelor of Science in Biology University of California Irvine Irvine, CA	2006-2009
Emergency Medical Technician – Paramedic Saddleback College Paramedic Program Mission Viejo, CA	2000-2001

HONORS & AWARDS

Alpha Omega Alpha Honor Medical Society University of California, Irvine School of Medicine Irvine, CA	2012-Present
Medical Student Teaching Award University of California, Irvine School of Medicine Irvine, CA	2012-2013
Phi Beta Kappa Honor Society University of California, Irvine Irvine, CA	2006-2009
Summa Cum-Laude Biological Sciences/Chemistry University of California, Irvine Irvine, CA	2006-2009
Excellence in Team Achievement Award Saddleback College Paramedic Program Mission Viejo, CA	2000-2001
Excellence in Pharmacology Award Saddleback College Paramedic Program Mission Viejo, CA	2000-2001

Example CV continued

JOHN DOE

PROFESSIONAL EXPERIENCE

Emergency Medical Technician – Paramedic 2004-2010
Lynch Ambulance
Anaheim, CA

Emergency Medical Technician – Basic 2001-2004
Care Ambulance Service
Orange, CA

CERTIFICATION & LICENSURE

Advanced Cardiac Life Support	2002-Present
Advanced Trauma Life Support	2002-2008
Pediatric Advanced Life Support	2002-2008
California State Paramedic License	2002-2008
Instructor, Basic Life Support	2002-2004

PROFESSIONAL ACTIVITIES

Instructor, Advanced Cardiac Life Support 2006-2010
Lynch Ambulance
Anaheim, CA

Paramedic Field Training Officer 2006-2010
Care Ambulance Service
Orange, CA

Instructor, Basic Life Support 2002-2004
Care Ambulance Services
Orange, CA

PROFESSIONAL MEMBERSHIPS

American College of Emergency Physicians	2010-Present
Emergency Medicine Residents' Association	2010-Present
American Medical Association	2010-Present

PERSONAL

Hobbies include winemaking, hiking, playing piano and singing.

student's personal statements over the years and found that they are becoming less and less "personal." Most medical students write about why they chose a particular specialty, how they enjoy the hands-on aspect of the specialty or their desire to comfort anxious patients. Unfortunately, there are no strong studies measuring the importance of the personal statement in regards to the overall application. Only 41% of the program directors that answered a survey looking at anesthesiology residency applications found personal statements to be very or somewhat important in selecting candidates for interviews. In a separate study, more than 90% of program directors used the personal statement during the actual interviews. Although the personal statement is not a critical piece to your overall application, it might give you an edge if you strike a chord with the reader.

Personal statements typically do not make or break your application. However, be careful how you word your personal statement. Plagiarism is an instant application killer. An Annals of Internal Medicine study found 5.2% of personal statements showed evidence of plagiarism. Avoid exaggerating your abilities or experiences as program directors may view this as dishonest.

Another application killer is poor grammar. One study reported more than 90% of program directors found the proper use of English to be a somewhat or very important feature of the essay. Make sure you have multiple people proof-read your essay. You have months to write your personal statement. Any error is considered unacceptable.

Letters of Recommendation

Letters of recommendation continue to be an important part of the application. In the 2013 NRMP Program Director Survey, 93% of program directors considered letters of recommendation in the specialty an important factor when selecting applicants to interview. In that same survey, letters of recommendation received a score of 4.8 out of 5 where 5 was considered very important in ranking applicants.

There has been tremendous controversy over the utility of the traditional narrative letter of recommendation. Many program directors have expressed frustrating comments like "all applicants appear the same," or "all are outstanding." The time required to read the letters was also an area of concern. As a result, the Council of Emergency Medicine Residency Directors task force (CORD) developed the Standardized Letter of Evaluation (SLOE), formerly known as Standardized Letter of Recommendation (SLOR).

A SLOE consists of background information on the applicant and letter writer, personal characteristics, global assessment and an open narrative section. A recent study found that both the background data and qualification data were predictive of success. Interestingly, an "outstanding" global assessment score and work ethic score were statistically predictive of a guaranteed match. However, another study found the global assessment score section to be an accurate predictor only 26% of the time.

As you can see, the SLOE is not an accurate predictor of your future. If you received an "outstanding" score you are still not home free. The best predictor for success is your desire and drive. When a program director reads your SLOE they should visualize the 9 P's (see chapter 2). Make sure your letter writer is familiar with the format. You can download it from cordem.org. Not all programs require letters to be in SLOE format. Most AOA residency programs accept the traditional narrative letter of recommendation.

In general, three to four letters of recommendation are sufficient. Make sure physicians that know you well write them. Generalized letters will add little value to your application. At least one letter (preferably two) should be from physicians in the specialty you are applying to. Ideally, you want each letter to discuss a different aspect of your character, personality, patient care, work ethic, how you fit into a specific program, etc.

Having a physician from a different specialty write you a letter is okay. Usually, letters from program directors, department chairs and medical directors carry more weight. Do not substitute a letter from someone that knows you well for another letter from a department chairperson you scarcely know. Doing so might omit specific examples of your personality and performance that program directors identify as predictors for success.

Asking someone to write a letter of recommendation for you is not easy. If you're lucky, he or she will offer to write one before you ask. If you're not lucky, try to follow these 5 steps:

1. Do not ask if you have any doubt about the quality of the letter the person will write. If they seem hesitant to write the letter, find someone else. You want to be confident the letter is stellar when you submit your application.
2. Timing is important. Do not ask for a letter in the middle of a cardiac arrest. Wait until the person is not distracted and has the time to provide you their complete attention. Make sure you give them the opportunity to say no. It will not be a very good letter if they feel they are being forced. Give them at least 3 to 4 weeks to complete the letter.
3. Act appreciative when asking for a letter.
4. If it has been a while since you last spoke with your potential letter writer, try jogging his or her memory by hinting at the talent/skill/quality they observed you doing. It may just end up in the letter.
5. Personally thank them for taking the time to write the letter.

Make sure you update the person that wrote the letter for you. Most physicians like to hear their efforts made a positive impact on your future. See the examples below for ideas on how to ask for a letter of recommendation.

Example 1:

Dr. Smith, I appreciate all your teaching points this month. I will be taking them with me when I apply to residency this September. Do you think you have time to write me a strong letter of recommendation?

Example 2:

Dr. Smith, thank you for your insight this month. I am applying to residency in September and was hoping you had time to write me a favorable letter of recommendation with particular comments on our time in the clinic aspirating joints?

Example 3:

Dr. Smith, I am applying to residency this September and was hoping you had time to write a strong letter of recommendation on my behalf? I appreciated your teaching points this month and believe a letter from you would be well receipted.

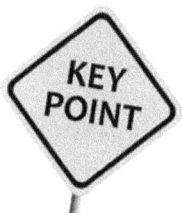

Start the application process early. It will allow you to identify areas of weakness and give you time to fill the gaps before you finalize your application

Chapter 5

The Interview

The most important part of the interview is staying true to your development plan and long term goals. By now you should have identified the 2 or 3 programs that align best with your plan. Do not schedule interviews for these 2 or 3 programs early in your interview plan. Your first few interviews provide you an opportunity to make mistakes but more importantly, learn interview dynamics. As you complete more and more interviews your comfort level improves and you will be more confident. During the last few interviews, you may begin to tire and lose interest. So, schedule the programs you value most in that sweet spot, somewhere in the mid to last half of your plan. The month in which you schedule your interview will not affect how you are ranked.

Do not schedule more than one interview per day. Most interviews will last several hours and include a hospital tour. A dinner the night before your interview is very common. Consider this your pre-interview interview. Schedule interviews for all the programs within the same geographic region together if possible. Traveling is expensive (plane ticket, rental car, hotel, gas, food, etc.). Having a credit card with saved frequent flyer miles is a plus. Now may be the time to cash in those miles. Spending three to five thousand dollars is common during interview season.

There are two parts to preparing for the interview. Part 1 is about knowing who you are and where you are going per your development plan. Part 2 is about knowing how the program can help you get there. Completing both will maximize your chances of success.

In Part 1, start by reviewing your long term goals. The interview panel cannot ask any surprise questions if you have a solid plan. For example, you already know why emergency medicine is right for you. Throughout your interviews you will be asked a wide range of questions. Answer them honestly and remember you can apply your professional plan to any question they ask. Also, look over your CV for potential interview questions on hobbies, board scores, GPA, research, work experience, etc. Spend time answering these questions to better prepare for interview day.

General questions:

1. What made you choose emergency medicine?

2. When did you know emergency medicine was right for you?
3. Where do you see yourself in 10 years?
4. What do you like most about emergency medicine and what do you like least about emergency medicine?
5. What specialty would you choose if you were not able to go into emergency medicine?
6. What would you do if you did not match?
7. Will you still be able to work as an emergency physician when you are in your 60's?
8. What are you looking for in a residency program?
9. Do you want to work in academic medicine or in the community setting when you finish residency?
10. Are you interested in completing a fellowship?
11. What is the biggest problem in emergency medicine right now?
12. Tell me about yourself?
13. What aspect of your CV do you want me to focus on and why?
14. What is your biggest strength and biggest weakness?
15. How would your friends describe you in one word?
16. Tell me about a time that you failed and what you learn from it?
17. Name a mistake that you made and how you

corrected it?
18. What was the hardest thing you have ever had to do?
19. Most challenging time in medical school?
20. Tell be about an Interesting case.
21. Talk about a time when you had to work with someone you disliked or did not get along with.
22. If you had a rack full of cases what type of case would you want to pick up?
23. How do you deal with stress?
24. What are your hobbies?
25. Favorite type of music?
26. Describe your role models?
27. What do you think will be the toughest aspect of emergency medicine for you?
28. There is a lot of information in your application; can you summarize your CV for me?
29. How do you define success?
30. What have you done that meets your definition of success?
31. If every program you applied to rank you as their number 1 candidate, what factors or considerations would you use to create your rank list?
32. What have you learned about yourself from your medical school experience?
33. What about our program attracted you to it?
34. How are you different from other candidates?
35. Suppose you are a resident and you have an

unmotivated medical student with you, how would you handle that situation?
36. How do you plan on balancing your professional and personal life?
37. What opportunities will you take advantage of if you come to our program?

Ethical Question:

A 35-year-old woman is rushed into the emergency department by EMS. The paramedic tells you she was in a major car accident and is severely bleeding. The woman is unable to talk. You order two units of packed red blood cells and tell the nurse to administer it right away. Just before the nurse starts the transfusion the patient's friend runs into the room and says, "Wait! She is a Jehovah's witness." The nurse turns to you and says, "Should I stop the transfusion?"

Obscure Questions:

1. If you were a kitchen appliance, which one would you be and why?
2. In volleyball, do you like rally scoring or serve scoring?
3. What is your fondest childhood memory?
4. Name the last book you read for fun?
5. What is your favorite meal?
6. What is the most adventurous thing you have ever done?
7. How would you spend 1 million dollars?

8. If you could have dinner with any three people dead or alive whom would they be and why?
9. Name three uses for a nasal cannula other than delivering oxygen?
10. How honest are you?

In Part 2, investigate the program's website. Look for any awards, accomplishments, future goals and identify the program's strengths and weaknesses. Find the program director, medical director, department chairs and faculty members and identify their accomplishments, goals, research and other areas of interests. Knowing what the interviewer is passionate about will help during the interview. Do not forget to look at the geography and local interests. Interviewers often compare your interests with local activities to gauge how happy you might be living in the area. You can use the information you obtain from the program's website during the interview. In fact, referencing the website demonstrates that you are a serious candidate. Be careful not to miss quote the website though and be prepared to discuss the topics you mention. If you discover any weaknesses during your internet search they can be used as questions at the end of the interview.

Arrive at the interview 30 to 45 minutes early. Give yourself plenty of time to use the restroom and get settled in before the interview. Showing up a few minutes before the interview start time is a warning to the program that you are irresponsible.

Dress appropriately. No obnoxious colors. No cartoon ties. Interviewing is serious business. Remember to bring copies of your CV.

Keep your composure during the interview even if your heart rate is 120 bpm. Maintain the appearance of being calm, cool and collected. Shake the interviewer's hand before and after the interview. If your hand is sweaty, wipe it across your pants before shaking their hand but do not be too obvious. Wait for the interviewer to take his seat before you sit down. Maintain good posture and keep eye contact. If the sun is shining right into your eyes, move. You want to be fully engaged in the interview. Do not chew gum. Do not curse. Do not mention any rumors you have heard about the program. Make sure you smile and above all else, be yourself.

There will undoubtedly be questions that are more difficult to answer than others. For example, can you explain why your board score is below average? It is important to stay calm when answering these types of questions. It is also important not to dwell on your answer or sound as if you are making excuses. Remember, one day does not make a career. Everyone has taken a bad exam at some point in their lives. Refocus the interviewers back to a particular part of your application that you excelled in and want to talk about. Your responses should always have a positive quality.

Make sure you have a few questions ready to ask the interview panel. You should consider your goals and what is important for you when developing questions. The more thought you put into the question the better the response. For example, if your goal is to practice international medicine, are there any opportunities to travel abroad? Alternatively, if you are interested in research, what type of support system does the program have for resident research? You can also visit the website of local news stations to see if any disasters have occurred in the area. Asking questions about financial stability, disaster planning, program goals and administration shows that you are evaluating the program critically and completely.

When the interview closes, you can ask for business cards or contact information. If you would like to return and spend time observing in the emergency department now is the time to ask. Many times, a few hours in the emergency department will clear up any lingering questions you still have about a program.

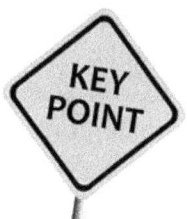

Staying true to your development plan and long term goals will enhance the value of the interview

Chapter 6

After the Interview

Write in your program interview log your likes and dislikes immediately after each interview. You will use this information to help prioritize programs on your rank list.

Make sure you have contact information on the residents, program coordinator and anyone else who interviewed you. Keeping in contact with the residents at the programs you are highly considering is important. Resident feedback was cited in 53% of programs as a factor involved in selecting candidates for interviews. The percentage for ranking candidates is likely to be similar. Sending emails, text messages and phone calls will keep you in the loop and could provide additional information about the program. As with everything, do not go overboard. One or two short emails or text messages over a four to five month period will be sufficient.

Be cautious when having conversations after the interview. Although it may sound like a program is highly interested in you, there are no commitments until the match has finalized. Strictly avoid conversations that discuss where a person/program is on the rank list. The NRMP has specific rules that must be met at all times. Report any violations. Do not make changes to your rank list based on post interview conversations.

Send a thank you letter to any program you are seriously considering. Do not send the same thank you letter to every program. Hand written letters are better than typed letters. If you send a letter to the individuals that interviewed you do not send the same letter to everyone. Try to personalize the letter by mentioning something you discussed during the interview. Your interview log can help. Also, make sure it is addressed to the right person. If you only send one letter to the program director keep the communication professional and clear. Thank you letters do not affect how a program will rank you. It is a professional courtesy. See the example letter for ideas.

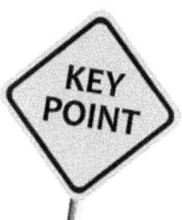

Post interview conversations are common. Keep them professional and do not let them impact your rank list

Example Thank You Letter

Hi Dr. _____,

I wanted to thank you again for the opportunity to interview at _____. The month I spent rotating at _____ was not only a very helpful and rewarding experience but also allowed me to examine the various EM programs. I enjoyed your program very much and it compares quite favorably to the other programs. The enthusiasm amongst the house staff, professional attitude, compassion, love of learning and camaraderie at _____ clearly results in a high level of patient care and satisfaction and aligns with what I want in the future.

I am excited to start my training and continue the same dedication to excellence that _____ strives to achieve.

I wish you and the _____ family a happy and safe new year.

Sincerely
_____, MSIV
School name
Address
Email address

Chapter 7

International Medical Graduate Considerations

I am constantly being asked, "How did you do it? What set you apart?" To fully answer these questions there are a number of different factors that need to be addressed including USMLE scores, Standardized letters of evaluation, programs, electives and Sub-Internships, research and applying. Before I discuss each of these it's important to understand the level of competition when applying to an emergency medicine residency. It is not my intent to scare you away from becoming an emergency physician; rather, I wish to inspire and motivate you by providing real world perspective on the uphill road you have ahead.

Successfully matching in emergency medicine is extremely difficult for international medical graduates (IMGs). The National Resident Matching Program and Educational Commission for Foreign Medical Graduates reported only 28% of U.S. IMGs matched to emergency medicine in 2013 while non-U.S. IMGs matched 37%. In the same report, the probability of matching to emergency medicine reached 90% if the total number of programs ranked was 17 for U.S. IMGs and 13 for non-U.S. IMGs. These totals far exceed the 8-10 needed by U.S. graduating medical students.

USMLE Scores

Most programs designate a minimum USMLE score, total number of repeat attempts due to failures and a litany of other criteria that must be met before an interview is offered. Unfortunately, there is no magic number for every program. The average USMLE Step 1 score for candidates that matched in 2013 was 225 for U.S. IMGs and 226 for non-U.S. IMGs. The average USMLE Step 1 score for candidates that did not match in 2013 was 215 for U.S. IMGs and 217 for non-U.S. IMGs. The majority of programs will set their minimum USMLE score above 200. Some programs will set their cutoff score at 220 while others will not designate a cutoff score. To meet the USMLE score cutoff for most programs keep your USMLE step 1 score well above 210. If you do not meet the USMLE score cutoff the likelihood that you will be granted an interview is low.

A strong USMLE score is an important part of

your application but does not guarantee a match. The probability of successfully matching to emergency medicine with a USMLE Step 1 score of 255 is 59% for non-U.S. IMGs and only 54% for U.S. IMGs. Unfortunately, many program directors will only overlook the IMG status if a candidate has a board score above 240. Researching each program before you apply will improve your chances of matching.

Performing well on a standardized test does not make you a good physician, let alone a good emergency physician. A well-rounded applicant with a good personality and excellent standardized letters of evaluation is considered highly competitive when compared to someone with fantastic USMLE scores, average standardized letters of evaluation and a bad attitude.

Standardized Letters of Evaluation

The program director, assistant program director or medical student clerkship director usually fills out the standardized letter of evaluation (SLOE) after they take into account your daily evaluations from the various faculty members . These letters are worth their weight in gold. They ask the evaluator specific questions that measure your level of performance relative to other applicants to provide an accurate description of your progress over the month long rotation. These SLOEs are extremely candid and honest and helps a program assess where you might rank on their list, if they were to rank you. You should have your SLOE written in emergency departments that have an emergency medicine residency since a significant number of questions pertain to where you would land on their rank list, if at all (see Chapter 4).

Electives and Sub-Internships

Obtaining an elective or Sub-Internship (Sub-I) can be a daunting experience for IMGs since they are unable to apply for rotations through the visiting student application service (VSAS). There are various programs that accept IMGs into residency but very few accept IMGs for electives or Sub-I's. This makes it even more difficult for IMGs to match into emergency medicine. Find the programs that matched IMGs within the last five years to identify possible locations for electives or Sub-I's. Then, contact these programs and ask if they allow IMGs to rotate in their department. Start this process early and make sure you have your work (or student) visa in order.

If you are able to schedule an elective or Sub-I you must perform well to be offered an interview and possibly match. Consider this rotation a month long interview. Your goal during this rotation is to outperform your U.S. counterparts and demonstrate why you deserve an opportunity to match. Spending one month at a specific site allows the program to see how you act when you are tired, hungry, stressed, on a night or early morning shift or being challenged with learning a new procedure. The program will also see how you interact with faculty, residents, nurses, technicians, secretaries and even the housekeeping staff. This information allows a program to better judge a candidate's suitability than a one-day interview. Most program directors will likely rank an applicant higher if he or she is well known and performs well. It is important to understand that emergency medicine is a "team sport." This means if a patient soils themselves and the nurses need help cleaning/changing the patient, do not walk out of the room thinking this is not a physician job. Taking care of the patient is your job. Spending five minutes helping the nurses will do wonders for the patient and prove to the nursing staff that you are a team player. However, if you have an attitude or develop a problem with the staff your rank will be affected.

Electives and Sub-I's are your opportunity to demonstrate why you should be considered for an interview. They also provide an opportunity to obtain a SLOE. If you are unable to schedule an elective or Sub-I or were only able to obtain one SLOE, your other letters should be regular letters of recommendation written by emergency physicians.

Research

Research improves your application and demonstrates an effort to better understand the evidence that clinicians use to treat patients. Although it does not make or break your application, it will be used as a talking point during your interview. For example, during one interview I was asked to explain a published article and my level of participation. During that interview, the program director said, "Many of the applicants who have their names on articles or publications have done little or no work and do not understand the topics or inner workings of the research." Make sure you understand the research projects you are involved in and be able to answer questions related to it. Otherwise, you will demonstrate a lack of commitment and poor work ethic which are red flags for program directors.

Applying

Before completing your ERAS application have someone you trust proofread your CV and personal statement for grammar, spelling and completeness (see Chapter 4). Do not put anything in your ERAS application, CV or personal statement that is not true or inaccurate. Honesty, trust and integrity are the hallmarks of being a physician. As an emergency physician, doing the right thing is important not only for the patient's survival but also for the physician's survival in the field. Remember, emergency medicine is an extremely small community. Exaggerating your experience can tarnish your reputation and prevent you from successfully matching.

Conclusion

The road to a successful match for IMGs is not easy. It requires determination, tenacity and hard work to overcome the odds stacked against you. Still, many IMGs successfully match every year and enjoy the honor and privilege of caring for patients during their most scary and critical moments. Understanding these odds and developing an action plan to overcome them is the best way to earn a resident position in emergency medicine (see Chapter 1).

Good luck to you and wish all the best in the upcoming match season.

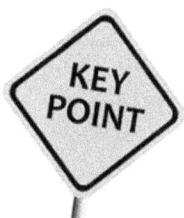

A successful match for IMGs requires planning, commitment and hard work

Chapter 8

Final Words

The best approach to a successful match is developing a plan with goals. Your plan serves as a foundation and roadmap that will guide you towards achieving your goals.

The list of potential residency programs is enormous. Choosing which program is right for you can be difficult and overwhelming. Having a plan will narrow your focus and help you create a more manageable list of programs.

Evaluating each program in measured fashion requires preparation and hard work. Remember, you will learn medicine no matter which program you chose. However, your level of happiness can depend on whether or not you had a plan and stayed true to that plan throughout the match process. So, be smart about your decision, as you will be spending the next three to five years of your life there and possibly more if you sign on as an attending after residency.

Rank the programs you love first and the

programs you like least last. Do not worry about where you think programs will rank you. The match process is designed to favor applicants opposed to the residency programs. If you would rather have your teeth pulled than go to a particular program do not rank it. You will be doing your colleagues and your patients a disservice if you are unhappy.

This is an exciting time in your professional development. You are finally able to take control of your future and explore opportunities within the specialty that interest you. Your goals may change as you mature and that is okay. Building on old experiences and creating new ones are part of life.

What you habitually think largely determines what you will ultimately become
— Bruce Lee

Congratulations on your continued success!

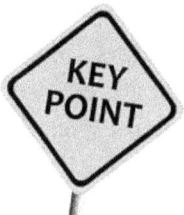

Following your developmental plan in a stepwise fashion is the best way to ensure a successful match

References:

1. DeSantis M, Marco CA. Emergency residency selection: factors influencing candidate decisions. Acad Emerg Med. 2005;12(6):559-561.
2. Laskey S, Cydulka KR. Applicant Considerations Associated with Selection of an Emergency Medicine Residency Program. Acad Emerg Med. 2009;16:355–359.
3. Crane JT, Ferraro CM. Selection criteria for emergency medicine residency applicants. Acad Emerg Med. 2000;7(1):54-60.
4. Groke Steven, et al. Evaluating applicants to a new emergency medicine residency program: subjective assessment of applicant characteristics. Int J Emerg Med. 2010;3(4):265-269.
5. Rasoul Mokabberi, et al. Immediate Impact of Participation in the Electronic Residency Application Service on a Fellowship Program. J Grad Med Educ. 2010;2(1):126-128.
6. Alfred St. Amour, Bruce. Factors Important to Applicants to Osteopathic Versus Allopathic Emergency Medicine Residency Programs. West J Emerg Med. 2013;15(2):184-187.
7. Leahy M, Cullen W, Bury G. "What makes a good doctor?" A cross sectional survey of public opinion. Ir Med J. 2003;96(2):38-41.

8. Yarris LM, Delorio NM, Lowe RA. Factors Applicants Value when Selecting an Emergency Medicine Residency. West J Emerg Med. 2009;10(3):159-162.
9. Lin, Michelle. Multiple Mini-Interview (MMI): Annals of EM Perspective article. Acad Life in Emerg Med. Web. 9 May 2014. (http://www.aliem.com/multiple-mini-interviews-annals-em-resident-perspective-article/).
10. Adams LJ, Brandenburg S, Blake M. Factors Influencing Internal Medicine Program Directors' Decisions about Applicants. J Assoc. Am Med Colleges. 2000;75(5):542-543.
11. Breyer MJ, Sadosty A, Biros M. Factors Affecting Candidate Placement on an Emergency Medicine Residency Program's Rank Order List. West J Emerg Med. 2012;13(6):458-462.
12. Wald DA, et al. The state of the clerkship: a survey of emergency medicine clerkship directors. Acad Emerg Med. 2007;14(7):629-634.
13. Katz B, Klauer K, James AG. So You Want a New Job: Time to Update Your CV. Boston Scientific Assembly. 2009. (http://acep.omnibooksonline.com/Boston2009/data/papers/MO-53.pdf).
14. White BA, et al. Is the evaluation of the personal statement a reliable component of the general surgery residency application? J

Surg Educ. 2012;69(3):340-343.
15. Carek PJ, et al. Recruitment behavior and program directors: how ethical are their perspectives about the match process? J Fam Med. 2000;32(4):258-260.
16. Max BA, et al. Have personal statements become impersonal? An evaluation of personal statements in anesthesiology residency applications. J Clin Anesth. 2010;22(5):346-351.
17. Segal S, et al. Plagiarism in residency application essays. Ann Intern Med. 2010;153(2):112-120.
18. Olson DP, et al. The Residency Application Abyss: Insights and Advice. Yale J Biol Med. 2011;84(3):195-202.
19. Kumwenda B, Dowell J, Husbands A. Is embellishing UCAS personal statements accepted practice in applications to medicine and dentistry? Med Teach. 2013;35(7):599-603.
20. DeZee KJ, et al. Letters of recommendation: rating, writing, and reading by clerkship directors of internal medicine. Teach Learn Med. 2009;21(2):153-158.
21. Keim SM, et al. A Standardized letter of recommendation for residency application. Acad Emerg Med. 1999;6(11):1141-1146.
22. Wagoner NE, Suriano JR, Stoner JA. Factors used by program directors to select residents. J Med Educ. 1986;61(1):10-21.
23. Stohl HE, Hueppchen NA, Bienstock JL.

The Utility of Letters of Recommendation in Predicting Resident Success: Can the ACGME Competencies Help? J Grad Med Educ. 2011;3(3):387-390.
24. Wright SM, Ziegelstein RC. Writing More Informative Letters of Reference. J Gen Intern Med. 2004;19(5 Pt 2): 588-593.
25. National Resident Matching Program, Data Release and Research Committee: Results of the 2012 NRMP Program Director Survey. National Resident Matching Program, Washington, DC. 2012.
26. National Resident Matching Program, Charting Outcomes in the Match, 2011. National Resident Matching Program, Washington, DC 2011.
27. Jena AB1, et al. The prevalence and nature of postinterview communications between residency programs and applicants during the match. Acad Med. 2012;87(10):1434-1442.
28. Martin-Lee L, Park H, Overton DT. Does interview date affect match list position in the emergency medicine national residency matching program match? Acad Emerg Med. 2000;7(9):1022-1026.
29. Yarris LM, Deiorio NM, Gaines SS. Emergency Medicine Residency Applicants' Perception about Being Contacted after Interview Day. West J Emerg Med. 2011;11(5):474-478.
30. Anderson KD, Jacobs DM, Blue AV. Is

match ethics an oxymoron? Am J Surg. 1999;177(3):237-239.
31. National Resident Matching Program. NRMP statement on professionalism communication. 2011.
32. Carek PJ, Anderson KD. Residency selection process and the match: does anyone believe anybody? JAMA. 2001;285:2784-2785.
33. Carek, Peter J. Postinterview Communications Between Residency Programs and Candidates: What are the Rules? J Grad Med Educ. 2012;4(2):263-264.
34. Association of American Medical College (AAMC). FACTS: Applicants, Matriculants, Enrollment, Graduates, MD/PhD, and Residency Applicants Data. Web. 2013. (https://www.aamc.org/data/facts/).
35. National Resident Matching Program and Educational Commission for Foreign Medical Graduates. Charting Outcomes in the Match for International Medical Graduates. 2014.

Notes:

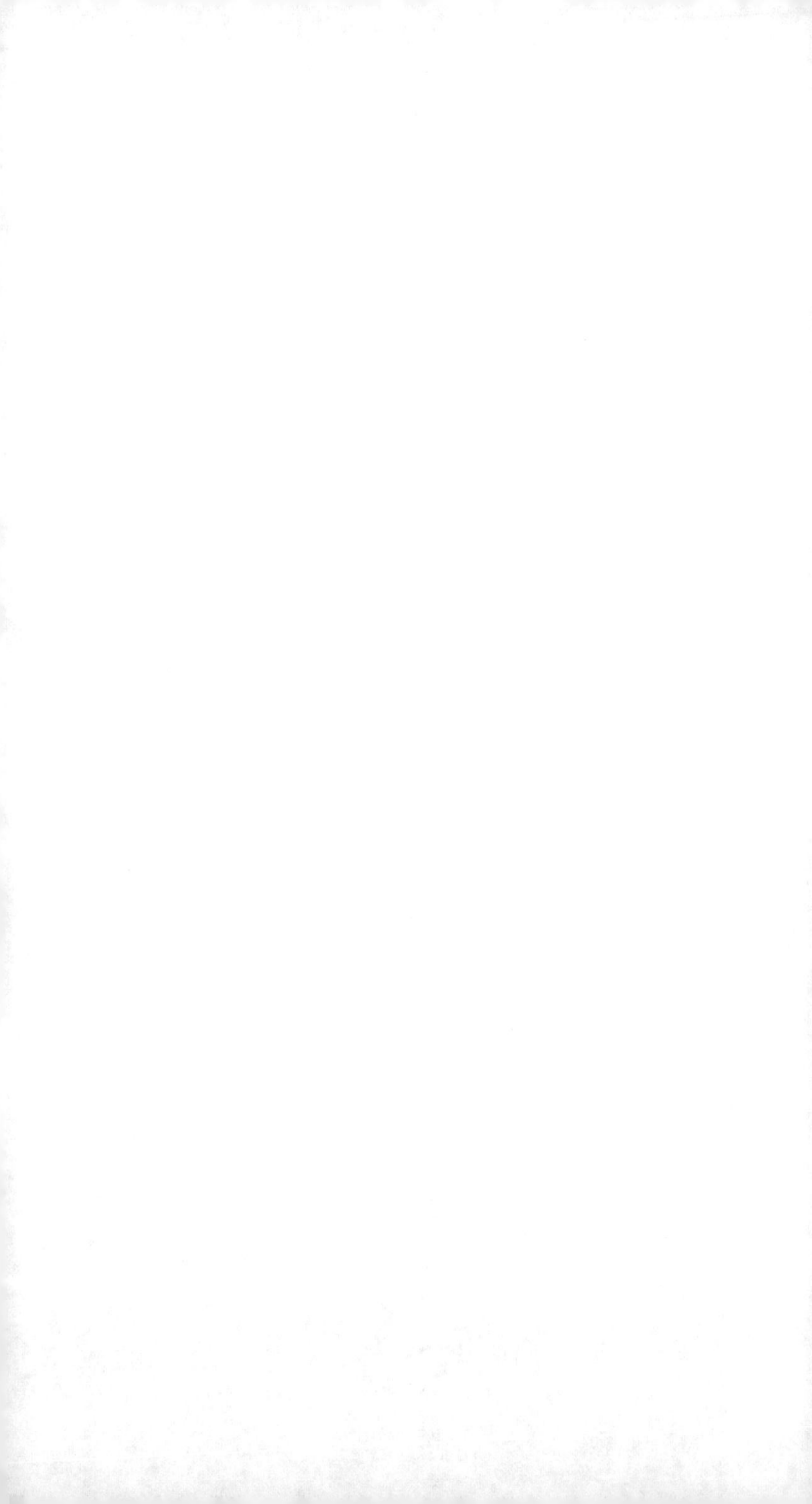

www.ingramcontent.com/pod-product-compliance
Lightning Source LLC
LaVergne TN
LVHW051202080426
835508LV00021B/2771